D1277516

MEDICARE INSURANCE

Simplified

(2020)

BY LINDA A. BELL

Medicare Insurance Simplified (2020)
by Linda A. Bell
NPN: #17973622

Website: HeartToHeartInsurance.com
Email: Linda@HeartToHeartInsurance.com

Medical/Medicaid & Medicare/Medicare insurance /Linda A. Bell
- 1st. ed.

ISBN-13: 9781074809188

Printed in the United States of America

DISCLAIMER

While every attempt has been made to provide accurate information in this book, the author, publisher, and Heart to Heart Insurance Agency LLC make no representations or warranties with respect to the accuracy or completeness of the contents of this work, and shall have neither liability nor responsibility to any person or entity with respect to any loss or damage caused or alleged to be caused directly or indirectly by the information contained herein, which is subject to change without notice. Please note that benefits, premiums, deductibles, copayments/coinsurance, provider networks, pharmacy networks, and/or formularies may change on January 1 of each year.

TABLE OF CONTENTS

PREFACE

Whenever I meet with someone who is turning 65 to talk about Medicare plans, I always ask if they clearly understand what Original Medicare Part A and Part B covers and doesn't cover, and how Part C, Part D, and Medigap plans help you fill some of the gaps in coverage to minimize your financial risk.

Most of them will shake their head, roll their eyes, and shout, "No! It's soooo confusing!" They feel overwhelmed by the complexity of this health insurance program.

Oftentimes, people are so afraid of making the wrong choice about their Medicare options, they make no choice at all, and simply have Part A and Part B coverage. They have no idea how financially vulnerable they are. A serious illness or injury that requires surgery and a lengthy hospital and rehab stay can potentially add up to a catastrophic amount of money, and there is NO LIMIT on Part A and Part B out-of-pocket costs if you have Original Medicare alone. But, we don't know what we don't know.

This is my *why*. It's why I became a licensed insurance agent. It's why I wrote this book. And it's why I designed a set of Medicare Insurance Simplified Flashcards™ and other materials for agents and educators.

My mission is to help you understand how Medicare works. This knowledge will empower you with the ability to make an informed decision about the type of Medicare coverage you'd like to have so you can choose a plan that fits your personal needs, preferences, and priorities — *and* protects you financially.

- From the heart, Linda A. Bell

MEDICARE IN A NUTSHELL

Let's start with a quick overview of some Medicare insurance basics.

Original Medicare (the plan that's administered by the federal government) has two parts: Part A and Part B.

This federal health insurance program is for people 65 years of age and older, people under 65 with a qualifying disability, and people of any age with End-Stage Renal Disease (ESRD), or Amyotrophic Lateral Sclerosis, also known as Lou Gehrig's Disease (ALS). To be eligible for coverage you must be a U.S. citizen or a permanent legal resident living in the United States for at least 5 years. This includes the 50 states, District of Columbia, Puerto Rico, U.S. Virgin Islands, Guam, Northern Mariana Islands, and American Samoa.

Part A is hospital (inpatient) insurance.

You can go to ANY hospital or other facility in the U.S. that accepts Medicare.
- **Part A covers** your inpatient hospital stay, skilled nursing care in a skilled nursing facility, home health care, and hospice care services.
- **Your cost for Part A** includes a monthly premium, hospital deductible, hospital coinsurance, and skilled nursing facility coinsurance.

Part B is medical (outpatient) insurance.

You can go to ANY doctor or other provider in the U.S. who accepts Medicare.

- **Part B covers** your medically necessary services, mental health care, preventative and screening services, and durable medical equipment.
- **Your cost for Part B** includes a monthly premium, annual deductible, medical copayment, and medical coinsurance.

There is NO LIMIT on out-of-pocket costs for those who are enrolled in Medicare Part A and Part B alone.

YOU HAVE A CHOICE.

Medicare insurance plans are also available through private insurance companies approved by Medicare.

Part C is a Medicare Advantage plan.
This is an all-in-one alternative to Original Medicare.
- **Part C provides** all of your Part A and Part B benefits. Plans are usually bundled with a Medicare Prescription Drug plan (Part D), plus extras.
- **Your cost for Part C** includes a monthly premium, annual deductible, copayment, and coinsurance.

All Medicare Advantage plans have a maximum out-of-pocket limit.

Part D is a Prescription Drug plan.
Often referred to as a PDP, these stand-alone drug plans may help you lower your prescription drug costs.
- **Part D covers** prescription drugs. Each plan has its own formulary, which is their list of covered drugs.
- **Your cost for Part D** includes a monthly premium, annual deductible, copayment, and coinsurance.

Medigap is a Medicare Supplement Insurance plan.

Medigap is an add-on supplemental policy for Original Medicare.

- **Medigap plans cover** some of the costs that Original Medicare doesn't pay for covered services and supplies, such as your copays, coinsurance, etc.
- **Your cost for a Medigap plan** varies by company.

There are currently (10) standard Medigap plans: **a, b, c, d, f, g, k, l, m**, and **n**.

"Why are there so many Medicare options? Isn't the Medicare plan that we get from the federal government good enough?"

Original Medicare insurance is very good, but it doesn't cover everything. There are many gaps in coverage, and the out-of-pocket costs associated with Medicare Part A and Part B can add up to *a lot of money*.

Now, let's dive in and take a closer look at how Medicare insurance works.

MEDICARE PART

A

ORIGINAL MEDICARE

HOSPITAL [INPATIENT] INSURANCE

PART A COVERS
INPATIENT HOSPITAL CARE

Medicare Part A covers your **INPATIENT HOSPITAL CARE** when a doctor admits you to a hospital that accepts Medicare to treat your illness or injury and all required conditions are met. This includes inpatient care in:

- **Acute care hospitals**
- **Critical access hospitals**
- **Long-term-care hospitals** that specialize in treating patients who are hospitalized for more than 25 days, such as those who used a ventilator for an extended period of time, experienced a severe wound or head injury, or have an ongoing medical condition that may not improve, like Alzheimer's Disease, Lou Gehrig's Disease (ALS), Multiple Sclerosis, Parkinson's Disease, or a stroke, and treatment is medically necessary to help prevent the condition from getting worse.
- **Psychiatric hospitals/psychiatric hospital units** Up to 190 days of inpatient care per lifetime.
- **Inpatient rehabilitation facilities**
- **Religious non-medical health care institutions** Covers only the non-religious, non-medical items and services associated with your inpatient care.

Inpatient hospital care includes (but may not be limited to): general nursing · meals · semi-private room · and other hospital services and supplies, including drugs received as part of your inpatient treatment.

PART A COVERS
SKILLED NURSING CARE IN A SKILLED NURSING FACILITY

Medicare Part A covers **SKILLED NURSING CARE PROVIDED IN A SKILLED NURSING FACILITY (SNF)** on a short-term basis if all required conditions are met, such as a 3-day minimum medically necessary inpatient hospital stay for a related illness or injury. Your doctor must certify that you need daily skilled care (such as intravenous fluids and medications, or physical therapy) which can only be provided, from a practical standpoint, when you are an inpatient of a skilled nursing facility.

Skilled nursing care in a SNF includes (but may not be limited to): ambulance transportation · dietary counseling · meals · medical social services · medical supplies and equipment used in the SNF · medications · physical and occupational therapy · semi-private room · skilled nursing care · speech-language pathology services · and swing bed services.

Medicare will not cover the cost of long-term care if "custodial" (non-medical) care is the only care you need, such as help getting dressed, bathing, etc.

Therefore, nursing home care is generally NOT covered by Medicare.

PART A COVERS
HOME HEALTH CARE

Medicare Part A covers eligible **HOME HEALTH CARE** services if you meet all of the conditions. A doctor, or a health care professional who works with your doctor, must see you face-to-face and certify that you need home health services because you have trouble leaving your home without help due to an illness or injury, and he/she recommends that you not leave home because of your condition. (You may be able to leave home for medical treatments or short, infrequent absences for non-medical reasons, such as attending religious services or adult daycare.)

Home health care includes (but may not be limited to): intermittent or part-time home health aide care · intermittent or part-time skilled nursing care · medical social services · occupational therapy · physical therapy · and speech-language pathology services.

PART A COVERS
HOSPICE CARE SERVICES

Medicare Part A covers **HOSPICE CARE SERVICES** to manage pain and symptoms related to a terminal illness if you meet all of the conditions. A hospice doctor and your doctor must certify that you are terminally ill and have a life expectancy of 6 months or less.

Hospice patients receive palliative care, which is care that's focused on keeping you comfortable, rather than to cure your illness.

Hospice care services include (but may not be limited to): counseling · doctor services · drugs for symptom control or pain relief · hospice aide and homemaker services · medical equipment and supplies · nursing care · pain and symptom management · physical and occupational therapy · short-term inpatient care to manage pain and symptoms · short-term respite care · and social services.

Inpatient vs. outpatient hospital status.

You are an **inpatient** if a doctor has written an order to formally admit you to the hospital. Your hospital stay is covered by Part A. Your last inpatient day is the day before you are discharged.

NOTE: If the doctor sends you to a skilled nursing facility for inpatient rehab care instead of releasing you to go home, Medicare will only cover the cost of your care if you've had a 3-day minimum, medically necessary inpatient hospital stay for a related illness or injury, along with other criteria.

If a doctor has *not* formally admitted you to a hospital or other facility you are an **outpatient**. Your X-rays, lab tests, outpatient surgeries, and medical emergency services are covered by Part B, even if you stay overnight in a hospital bed "under observation."

The hospital is required to give anyone who receives outpatient observation services for more than 24 hours a Medicare Outpatient Observation Notice that will explain why you are getting outpatient observation services, and how this may affect the cost of your hospital care and any other care you get after leaving the hospital.

YOUR COST

MEDICARE PART A

HOSPITAL [INPATIENT] INSURANCE

YOUR COST FOR PART A (2020)

MONTHLY PREMIUM

If you (or your spouse) worked and paid Medicare taxes for:	
40 or more quarters	**$0/month**
30-39 quarters	**$252/month**
Less than 30 quarters	**$458/month**

Most people don't pay a monthly premium. (You've essentially paid this premium in advance. 40 quarters is the equivalent of ten or more years.)

Part A late-enrollment penalty

If you are not eligible for premium-free Part A, and you don't enroll in Part A when you're first eligible for coverage, you may pay a 10% higher premium for twice the number of years that you could've had Part A, but didn't.

YOUR COST FOR PART A (2020)

HOSPITAL DEDUCTIBLE

$1,408
for inpatient services.

This is the amount you must pay per benefit period before Medicare will begin to pay for your hospital inpatient services.

A benefit period begins the day you are formally admitted to the hospital (or skilled nursing facility) by a doctor as an inpatient; it ends when you have received NO inpatient hospital (or skilled care in a skilled nursing facility) for 60 days in a row.

NOTE: There's NO LIMIT to the number of benefit periods a person can have in their lifetime. *It's possible to have as many as six benefit periods in one year!*

Potential financial risk:

$1,408 hospital deductible x
6 possible benefit periods
= $8,448

YOUR COST FOR PART A (2020)

HOSPITAL COINSURANCE

Days 1-60	**$0/day**
Days 61-90	**$352/day**
(60) Lifetime reserve days*	**$704/reserve day**
After that	**You pay 100%**

This is your share of the cost for hospital inpatient care per benefit period after you've paid the hospital deductible.

*Medicare gives you 60 reserve days (maximum per lifetime) to use after a 90-day hospital stay. When these are gone you pay 100% of the cost for your hospital stay after 90 days.

Potential financial risk per benefit period:

Days 61-90 (30 days) @ $352/day = $10,560

60 Lifetime Reserve days @ $704/day = $42,240

100% after that!

YOUR COST FOR PART A (2020)

SKILLED NURSING FACILITY COINSURANCE

Days 1-20	**$0/day**
Days 21-100	**$176/day**
After that	**You pay 100%**

This is your share of the cost for inpatient care in a skilled nursing facility per benefit period if your doctor transferred you there and you meet all of the criteria for coverage.

Potential financial risk per benefit period:

Days 21-100 (80 days) @ $176/day = $14,080

100% after that!

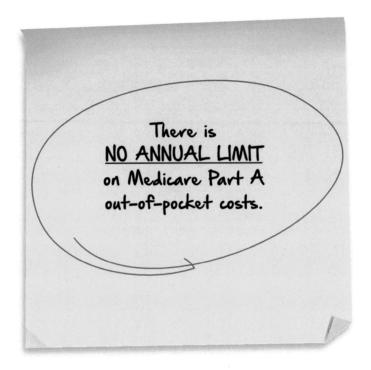

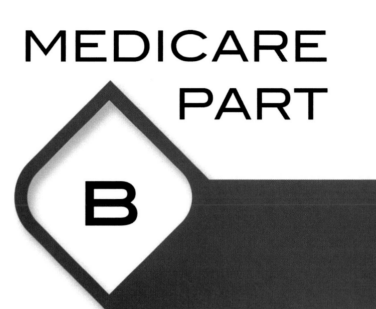

PART B COVERS
MEDICALLY NECESSARY SERVICES

Medicare Part B covers **MEDICALLY NECESSARY SERVICES** or supplies that are needed to diagnose or treat your medical condition and that meet accepted standards of medical practice. This includes visits to doctors, specialists, and other health care providers who accept Medicare assignment.

Medically necessary services include (but may not be limited to): ambulance services · clinical lab services · diagnostic tests · doctor and other health care provider services, including those received while you're in a hospital · outpatient hospital services · and second surgical opinion.

PART B COVERS

MENTAL HEALTH CARE

Medicare Part B covers **MENTAL HEALTH CARE** services including visits to doctors, specialists, and other health care providers who accept Medicare assignment. It also covers medically necessary services and supplies to diagnose or treat your mental health condition.

Mental health care includes (but may not be limited to): family counseling, if needed for your treatment · individual and group psychotherapy · medication management · treatment of inappropriate alcohol & drug use · partial hospitalization · psychiatric evaluation · and some prescription drugs, such as injections.

PART B COVERS
PREVENTATIVE & SCREENING SERVICES

Medicare Part B covers **PREVENTATIVE & SCREENING SERVICES** to prevent illness or detect it at an early stage. If you receive services from a health care provider who accepts Medicare assignment, you pay nothing for *most* of these services.

Preventative & screening services include (but may not be limited to): abdominal aortic aneurysm · alcohol misuse · bone density · cardiovascular disease · cervical & vaginal cancer · colorectal cancer · depression · diabetes · glaucoma · hepatitis B & C · HIV · lung cancer · mammograms · nutrition therapy · obesity · prostate cancer · sexually transmitted infections · shots (e.g., flu, hepatitis B, pneumococcal) · tobacco-use cessation · "Welcome to Medicare" (one-time visit) · and yearly "Wellness" visit.

PART B COVERS
DURABLE MEDICAL EQUIPMENT

Medicare Part B covers medically necessary **DURABLE MEDICAL EQUIPMENT** prescribed by a doctor for home care.

Durable medical equipment includes (but may not be limited to): air fluidized beds · blood sugar monitors and test strips · canes & crutches · CPM machine · hospital beds · infusion pumps & supplies · manual wheelchairs and power mobility devices · nebulizers · nebulizer medications · oxygen equipment & accessories · patient lifts · sleep apnea and continuous positive airway pressure (CPAP) devices & accessories · suction pumps · traction equipment · and walkers.

Medicare does NOT cover:
> Routine dental services or dentures
> Routine eye exams for glasses
> Routine foot care
> Routine preventative physical exams
> Acupuncture
> Cosmetic surgery
> Hearing exams for hearing aids
> Medical care while traveling outside the USA (with rare exceptions)
> Outpatient prescription drugs

YOUR COST

MEDICARE PART

B

MEDICAL [OUTPATIENT] INSURANCE

YOUR COST FOR PART B (2020)

MONTHLY PREMIUM

$144.60/month
Higher-income consumers may pay more.

This is the amount most people pay for their Part B monthly premium.

Part B late-enrollment penalty

If you don't enroll in Medicare Part B when you're first eligible for coverage, your monthly premium may go up 10% of the standard premium for each 12-month period that you could've had Part B, but didn't. *This is a lifelong penalty.*

YOUR COST FOR PART B (2020)

ANNUAL DEDUCTIBLE

$198/year
for outpatient services.

This is the amount you must pay before Medicare will begin to pay for your medical outpatient services.

YOUR COST FOR PART B (2020)

MEDICAL COPAYMENT

Typically a dollar amount
for outpatient services.

There's generally a copayment for each service you receive in a hospital outpatient setting (other than certain preventative services). In most cases, this copayment cannot exceed the amount of the Part A hospital deductible, unless the services were provided in a Critical Access hospital. So, if a doctor charges a higher fee to provide an outpatient service in a hospital than he/she would charge to provide the *same service* in his/her office, the fee will be capped at the Part A hospital deductible amount, which is $1,408 in 2020.

NOTE: A doctor, provider, or supplier who "accepts Medicare assignment" has signed an agreement with Medicare to accept the Medicare-approved amount for covered services as payment in full. A "non-participating" doctor, provider, or supplier has NOT signed an agreement to accept Medicare assignment, but may be willing to accept assignment for individual patients on a case-by-case basis. They may require you to pay the entire bill at the time of service. In some states, doctors who do not accept Medicare assignment can add an Excess Charge of up to 15% over and above the Medicare-approved amount for covered medical services.

YOUR COST FOR PART B (2020)

MEDICAL COINSURANCE

> ### Typically 20%
> of the Medicare-approved amount.

After your annual deductible is met, this is the amount you pay for most doctor services (including services you receive in the hospital from doctors, specialists, surgeons, etc., while you are a hospital inpatient), durable medical equipment, and Medicare Part B drugs, such as chemotherapy.

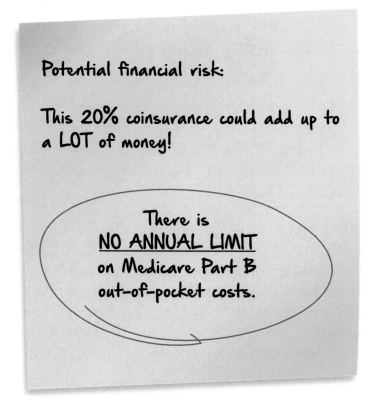

Potential financial risk:

This 20% coinsurance could add up to a LOT of money!

There is
NO ANNUAL LIMIT
on Medicare Part B
out-of-pocket costs.

PART A & PART B ENROLLMENT PERIODS

You can only enroll in or make a change to your Medicare coverage during specific enrollment periods.

Initial Enrollment Period (IEP)

You have a 7-month window of time to enroll in Medicare Part A and Part B for the first time. It begins 3 months before the month you turn 65, includes the month you turn 65, and ends 3 months after the month you turn 65.

For example, if your birthday is April 20th, you have from January 1st through July 31st to enroll in Medicare for the first time.

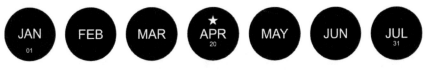

The best time to enroll is during the 3-month period before your birthday so your coverage can go into effect on the first day of the month in which you turn 65. (If your birthday is on the 1st day of the month, your coverage starts on the first day of the prior month.)

IF YOU ARE RECEIVING SOCIAL SECURITY BENEFITS when you turn 65, you will be automatically enrolled in Original Medicare. Your red, white, and blue Medicare ID card will arrive in the mail about three months before your 65th birthday. Your Medicare Part A and Part B effective dates will be printed on your card. (NOTE: If you live in Puerto Rico you must sign up for Part B; you won't get it automatically.)

IF YOU ARE NOT RECEIVING SOCIAL SECURITY BENEFITS when you are close to 65, you must enroll yourself in Medicare 3 months before your 65th birthday. An easy way to do this is to go to the Social Security website. (See: "my Social Security" and "Medicare Enrollment.") NOTE: If you have a fraud alert or you've put a freeze on your credit report, you may need to call EQUIFAX at 888-548-7878 and ask them to lift the freeze *before* you complete the online application. Otherwise, they won't be able to validate your identity and you'll have to drive over to your local Social Security office to apply for benefits in person.

IF YOU HAVE A DISABILITY AND YOU ARE UNDER 65, you'll be automatically enrolled in Part A and Part B after you have received Social Security benefits, or certain disability benefits from the Railroad Retirement Board, for 24 months.

IF YOU HAVE ALS (LOU GEHRIG'S DISEASE) your Medicare coverage starts immediately upon collecting Social Security Disability benefits.

IF YOU HAVE ESRD (END-STAGE RENAL DISEASE) your coverage generally starts 3 months after a course of regular dialysis begins or after a kidney transplant.

Should I delay my Part B enrollment?

If you or your spouse are still *actively* working when you turn 65, or if you have other insurance coverage contact benefits administrator before you turn 65 to find out how your insurance works with Medicare. In some cases, you may need to enroll in Part A and Part B to keep your coverage. In other cases, it may be better to delay your Part B enrollment.

IF YOU (OR YOUR SPOUSE) WORK FOR A COMPANY WITH LESS THAN 20 EMPLOYEES you MUST enroll in both Medicare Part A and Part B during your Initial Enrollment Period. According to the Medicare Secondary Payer Act, in this situation Medicare will automatically become your primary insurer when you turn 65 and your group health plan will be secondary. (An exception to this rule would be if the employer is part of a multiple or multi-employer group in which at least one employer employs 20 or more individuals.)

If you miss your Initial Enrollment Period and enroll in Part B during the GENERAL ENROLLMENT PERIOD (JAN 1 - MAR 31), your coverage won't start until JULY 1. This puts you at risk of having a lapse in coverage! Your secondary (employer) insurance may not pay on any claims if there is no primary insurer to process the claims first. You may also incur a lifelong Part B late enrollment penalty.

IF YOU (OR YOUR SPOUSE) WORK FOR A COMPANY WITH 20 OR MORE EMPLOYEES your group health plan is your primary insurer and Medicare is secondary. You should enroll in Medicare Part A during your Initial Enrollment Period if you qualify for premium-free Part A, as this may save you money if you are hospitalized. However, as a general rule, you should delay your Part B enrollment until you (or your spouse) stop working or lose your employer coverage; whichever comes first. This will save you from paying a monthly premium for a secondary insurance plan that only pays 80% of the Medicare-approved amount for Medicare-covered outpatient services *after* you've met the annual deductible. It will also enable you to postpone your 6-month Medigap Open Enrollment Period, which is triggered automatically when a person who is 65 or older enrolls in Part B.

If you are considering staying in Original Medicare and picking up a Medigap plan after you retire, it's vital for you to save this 6-month Medigap Open Enrollment Period until you're ready to enroll in a plan! During your (one-time) Medigap Open Enrollment Period, you are *guaranteed* to be covered, and at the same rate as a healthy person, even if you have a pre-existing health condition. After this enrollment period has passed, you may be required to go through medical underwriting to determine your insurability. You could be declined, have a waiting period, and/or pay a higher premium than other people unless you qualify for a Medigap Special Enrollment Period or your state doesn't allow medical underwriting of Medigap plans.

NOTE: To delay your Part B enrollment you must opt-out *before* your Medicare coverage begins. **DO NOT permanently cancel Part B;** just delay your enrollment. Call Medicare or the Social Security office a few months before you turn 65. Let them know that you are still actively working and ask how the Part B coverage pertains to your specific employment situation. They'll give you instructions on what to do.

General Enrollment Period (GEP)
JAN 1 - MAR 31

If you did not enroll in Medicare Part A and/or Part B when you were first eligible, and you are not eligible for a Special

Enrollment Period (SEP), you may enroll during this election period. Coverage starts JULY 1. *A lifelong late enrollment penalty may apply.*

Special Circumstances | Special Enrollment Periods (SEP)

When certain life events happen after your Initial Enrollment Period has passed you may be able to use a Special Enrollment Period to enroll in Medicare Part A and/or Part B. For example, if you or your spouse are *currently* working, and you are covered by a group health plan through the employer or union based on that work, you have an **8-month Special Enrollment Period** to enroll in Part A and/or Part B that starts:

- The month after the employment ends, OR
- The month after the group health insurance plan that's *based on your current employment* ends; whichever happens first.

NOTE: If you have a disability and your group health plan coverage is based on the current employment of a family member, the employer must have 100 or more employees for you to qualify for a Special Enrollment Period.

To enroll in Part A, you must contact your local Social Security office. To enroll in Part B, you must complete and send these two forms to your local Social Security office:

1. *"Application for Enrollment in Medicare Part B"* [CMS-40B]
2. *Request for Employment Information"* [CMS-L564E] (After you fill out Section A, have the employer fill out Section B and return it to you.)

COBRA does **NOT** meet the definition of coverage based on "current" employment.

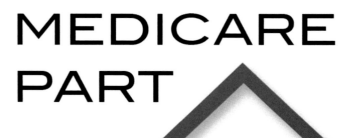

MEDICARE PART C

AVAILABLE THROUGH PRIVATE COMPANIES

MEDICARE ADVANTAGE PLAN

PART C: MEDICARE ADVANTAGE PLAN

Medicare Advantage is an all-in-one *alternative* to Original Medicare. (It is not a Medicare supplement.) The federal government pays private insurance companies to manage the care for each member, and cover almost all of the medically necessary services that Medicare Part A and Part B cover. (Original Medicare covers the cost of hospice care, some new Medicare benefits, and some cost for clinical research.) These plans must follow the rules set by Medicare.

To be eligible for a Medicare Advantage plan you must have Medicare Part A *and* Part B, and live in the plan's service area. You cannot have End-Stage Renal Disease (some exceptions apply), and you cannot be incarcerated. If you have employer or union health insurance coverage, enrolling in a Medicare Advantage plan could cause you and your dependents to lose your coverage, and you may not be able to get it back. Call your benefits provider before you enroll in a plan!

All Medicare Advantage plans have a maximum out-of-pocket limit, and will cover emergency and urgently needed medical care everywhere in the U.S. and its territories. Most plans are bundled with a Medicare Prescription Drug plan (Part D) plus other health and wellness programs. Benefits, formulary, pharmacy network, provider network, premium and/or copayments/coinsurance may change on January 1 of each year.

There are (6) types of Medicare Advantage plans.

Health Maintenance Organization (HMO)

In most HMO plans, you can only go to doctors, other health care providers, or hospitals that are in the plan's network. You may need a referral from your primary care doctor to visit other doctors and specialists, or to have medically necessary tests.

HMO Point-Of-Service (HMO-POS)

This type of HMO plan allows you to get some services out-of-network, usually for a higher copayment or coinsurance.

Medical Savings Account (MSA)

MSA plans have a very high annual deductible; it varies by company and plan. Medicare will deposit money into a special type of savings account to help you pay for your health care costs until you've met the deductible.

Preferred Provider Organization (PPO)

In a PPO plan, you can go to doctors, hospitals, and other health care providers outside of the plan's network, generally for a higher cost.

Private Fee-For-Service (PFFS)

Each PFFS plan specifies how much the doctors, other health care providers, and hospitals will get paid, and what you must pay for out-of-pocket. You can generally go to any doctor or other health care provider or hospital who will accept the plan's payment terms.

Special Needs Plan (SNP)

These plans provide benefits, services, provider choices, and drug formularies that are tailored to meet the needs of people with specific diseases, certain health care needs, or limited incomes.

PART C
PROVIDES ALL OF YOUR PART A BENEFITS

This includes:

INPATIENT HOSPITAL CARE

SKILLED NURSING CARE IN A SKILLED NURSING FACILITY

HOME HEALTH CARE

HOSPICE CARE SERVICES*

Original Medicare covers the cost for hospice care services.

PART C
PROVIDES ALL OF YOUR PART B BENEFITS

This includes:

MEDICALLY NECESSARY SERVICES*

MENTAL HEALTH CARE

PREVENTATIVE & SCREENING SERVICES

DURABLE MEDICAL EQUIPMENT

Original Medicare covers some new Medicare benefits, and some costs for clinical research studies.

PART C

USUALLY INCLUDES
PART D

Medicare Prescription Drug plans have 4 stages of coverage:

STAGE 1:
ANNUAL DEDUCTIBLE

STAGE 2:
INITIAL COVERAGE

STAGE 3:
COVERAGE GAP

STAGE 4:
CATASTROPHIC COVERAGE

Some Medicare Advantage plans
do not include prescription drug coverage.

PART C

USUALLY INCLUDES EXTRA BENEFITS

For example:

ROUTINE DENTAL CARE

ROUTINE EYE CARE

ROUTINE HEARING CARE

OTHER HEALTH & WELLNESS PROGRAMS

Extra benefits vary by company and plan.
Some plans may charge an extra fee for extra benefits.

Annual Notice of Changes | Evidence of Coverage

In the fall, your plan will send you a printed **Annual Notice of Changes (ANOC)** about changes to your Medicare Advantage plan's coverage, costs, service area, and more that will go into effect on JAN 1. Your plan will also send you an **Evidence of Coverage (EOC) notice or printed copy** that gives you details about what your plan covers, how much you pay, and more. Review these two notices carefully to make sure your plan will still meet your needs in the coming year. If not, you may switch plans during the Annual Enrollment Period (OCT 15 - DEC 7).

Star ratings

Medicare uses a star rating to measure the quality and performance of Medicare Advantage plans. The overall rating of a plan that covers health services tells you about the plan's quality in five areas:

1. Staying healthy (screening tests and vaccines)
2. Managing chronic (long-term) conditions
3. Member experience with the health plan
4. Member complaints and changes in the health plan's performance
5. Health plan customer service

This information is collected from:
- Member surveys
- Information that clinicians submit to Medicare
- Information that plans submit to Medicare
- Medicare's regular monitoring activities

If the plan covers prescription drugs too, the overall rating tells you about the drug plan's quality and performance as well. (See: star ratings for Medicare Prescription Drug plans.)

YOUR COST

MEDICARE PART C

MEDICARE ADVANTAGE PLAN

YOUR COST FOR PART C (2020)

MONTHLY PREMIUM

Varies
by company and plan.

Some insurance companies offer a Medicare Advantage plan with a $0/monthly premium, and some plans have a Part B premium reduction benefit, called a Part B Premium Give-Back. (These plans may not be available in all service areas.)

NOTE: You must continue to pay your Medicare Part B premium, even if the Medicare Advantage plan premium is $0.

YOUR COST FOR PART C (2020)

PLAN DEDUCTIBLE(S)

Varies
by company and plan.

This is the amount you must pay before the plan will begin to pay for your inpatient medical services, outpatient medical services, and/or prescription drugs.

YOUR COST FOR PART C (2020)

COPAYMENT & COINSURANCE

Varies
by company and plan.

After your annual deductibles have been met, this is the amount you pay for inpatient, outpatient, and prescription drugs, if they are included in your Medicare Advantage plan.

YOUR COST FOR PART C (2020)

MAXIMUM OUT-OF-POCKET LIMIT

HMO, HMO-POS (In-Network)	$6,700
PFFS (Non-Network, Combined)	$6,700
PPO (In-Network)	$6,700
PPO (Combined)	$10,000

All Medicare Advantage plans have a maximum out-of-pocket limit. The annual MOOP varies depending on the type of Medicare Advantage plan you are enrolled in, and whether all of your doctors and providers are in-network or a combination of in-network and out-of-network.

Some plans may choose to establish **lower annual limits.**

PART C
ENROLLMENT PERIODS

You can only enroll in, or make a change to, a Medicare Advantage plan (Part C) during specific enrollment periods.

Initial Coverage Election Period (ICEP)

IF YOUR PART A AND PART B HAVE THE SAME EFFECTIVE DATE you can enroll in a Medicare Advantage plan during your 7-month Initial Enrollment Period (IEP).

IF YOUR PART A AND PART B HAVE DIFFERENT EFFECTIVE DATES because you enrolled in one or the other during a Special Enrollment Period or the General Enrollment Period, your Initial Coverage Election Period (ICEP) begins 3 months before the effective date of whichever plan you added last; usually Part B. You have until the last day of the month before your coverage starts to enroll in a Medicare Advantage plan.

IF YOU ARE NEWLY ELIGIBLE FOR MEDICARE BECAUSE YOU HAVE A DISABILITY AND YOU ARE UNDER 65 you may enroll in a Medicare Advantage plan after you've received Social Security or Railroad Retirement Board (RRB) disability benefits for a full 24 months. You have 7 months to enroll in a plan. (Starts 3 months before your 25th month, includes the 25th month, and ends 3 months after your 25th month.) If you enroll during the 3 months before your 25th month, your coverage starts on the first day of the 25th month. If you enroll in the 25th - 28th month, your coverage starts on the first day of the month after you enroll.

IF YOU ARE ALREADY ELIGIBLE FOR MEDICARE BECAUSE YOU HAVE A DISABILITY AND YOU TURN 65 you may use your (7-month) Initial Enrollment Period (IEP) to:
- Enroll in a Medicare Advantage plan.
- Switch from your current Medicare Advantage plan to another Medicare Advantage plan.
- Drop your Medicare Advantage plan and return to Original Medicare; you may add a Medicare Prescription Drug plan (Part D).

12-month Medicare Advantage Trial Period: If you enroll in a Medicare Advantage plan when you are first eligible for coverage at age 65, you can drop your plan and return to Original Medicare at any time prior to the one-year anniversary of the effective date, and may add a Medicare Prescription Drug plan (Part D) to your coverage. You retain your Medigap Guaranteed Issue Rights during this trial period.

Annual Enrollment Period (AEP) OCT 15 - DEC 7

During this enrollment period, you may:
- Enroll in a Medicare Advantage plan.
- Switch from one Medicare Advantage plan to another Medicare Advantage plan.
- Drop your Medicare Advantage plan and return to Original Medicare; you may add a Medicare Prescription Drug plan (Part D).

Changes go into effect on JAN 1.

Medicare Advantage Open Enrollment Period (MA-OEP) JAN 1 - MAR 31

During this time you can make a one-time change:
- Switch from one Medicare Advantage plan to another Medicare Advantage plan.

- Drop your Medicare Advantage plan and return to Original Medicare; you may add a Medicare Prescription Drug plan (Part D) to your coverage.

Changes start on the first day of the month after the plan gets your request.

Medicare Advantage Open Enrollment Period: New (MA-OEP New)

New Medicare beneficiaries who enroll in a Medicare Advantage plan during their Initial Enrollment Period are entitled to a **3-month Medicare Advantage Trial Period.** During this time, you can make a one-time change to:

- Switch from one Medicare Advantage plan to another Medicare Advantage plan.
- Drop your Medicare Advantage plan and return to Original Medicare; you may add a Medicare Prescription Drug plan (Part D).

Special Circumstances | Special Enrollment Periods (SEP)

When certain life events happen after your Initial Coverage Election Period (ICEP) has passed, you may be able to use a Special Enrollment Period to enroll in, switch, or drop a Medicare Advantage plan. For example, you have a **2-month Special Enrollment Period** after leaving coverage from your employer or union.

5-Star Special Enrollment Period (5-Star SEP) DEC 8 - NOV 30

If a 5-Star Medicare Advantage plan, 5-Star Cost plan, or a 5-Star Medicare Prescription Drug plan is available in your service area, you can use this Special Enrollment Period to make a one-time switch to that plan. (A 5-star rating is considered excellent; these ratings can change every year.)

MEDICARE PART

D

AVAILABLE THROUGH PRIVATE COMPANIES

MEDICARE PRESCRIPTION DRUG PLAN

PART D:
PRESCRIPTION DRUG PLAN

Original Medicare does *not* cover outpatient prescription drugs. Stand-alone Medicare Prescription Drug plans (Part D) are available through private insurance companies. They may help to lower your prescription drug costs and protect you from price increases by locking in your cost for a full calendar year. Plans must follow rules set by Medicare.

To be eligible for Medicare Part D, you must be enrolled in Medicare Part A *or* Part B and live in the plan's service area. You cannot be incarcerated. If you have group health insurance coverage through your employer or union, enrolling in a Part D could cause you and your dependents to lose your coverage, and you may not be able to get it back. Call your benefits provider before you enroll in a plan!

Drug plans are required to give at least a standard level of coverage set by Medicare. They must cover both generic and brand-name prescription drugs; at least 2 drugs per drug category. Each plan decides which pharmacies they will use, which prescription drugs they will cover, and how much they will charge for their drugs. If your plan has preferred pharmacies, you may save money by using them.

Most plans group their drugs into cost-sharing tiers. For example, Tier 1: common generics, Tier 2: preferred brand-name drugs, Tier 3: non-preferred brand-name drugs, Tier 4: specialty (high-cost) drugs. Not all plans structure their tier levels in the same way; some plans have additional tiers. Plans are permitted to make changes to their formulary, such as to add or remove a drug, as long as they follow the guidelines set by Medicare.

Before you enroll in a Medicare Prescription Drug plan, check the formulary carefully to make sure all of your prescription drugs are covered. Depending on which prescription drugs you take, your out-of-pocket costs can vary significantly from plan to plan, so it's wise to shop around and compare plans. Benefits, formulary, pharmacy network, provider network, premium and/or copayments/coinsurance may change on January 1 of each year.

Formulary exceptions

If a formulary does not include a specific drug that you take, a similar drug should be available. In the event that you or your doctor believe that none of the drugs on your plan's formulary will work for your condition, you can request a formulary exception. If approved, the plan will cover that particular drug. In most cases, you must first try a certain less-expensive drug on the plan's formulary before you move up to a more expensive drug. This is called step therapy. Your prescriber can request an exception to this rule if you meet certain criteria.

Drugs you get in a hospital outpatient setting

In most cases, self-administered drugs (ones that you would normally take on your own) that are received while you have an outpatient status in a hospital setting, such as when you are "under observation" in an emergency room, are not covered by Part B. You will likely need to pay out-of-pocket for these. If you submit a claim to your drug plan they *may* cover these drugs and send you a refund.

Part D has 4 stages of coverage.

PART D COVERS

STAGE 1:
ANNUAL DEDUCTIBLE

In stage 1, which starts at the beginning of every calendar year, you must pay for your prescription drugs in full until you meet your plan's annual deductible amount.

If your Medicare Prescription Drug plan has no annual deductible, your coverage begins with Stage 2.

PART D COVERS

STAGE 2:
INITIAL COVERAGE

After you've met your annual deductible, you and the drug plan share the cost of covered drugs.

In stage 2, you will either pay a copayment (dollar amount) or a coinsurance (percentage of the plan's negotiated cost for prescription drugs).

PART D COVERS

STAGE 3: COVERAGE GAP

Your plan may have a gap in coverage, which is often referred to as *the donut hole,* if the amount of your year-to-date total drug cost reaches **$4,020.** If it does, you will enter Stage 3 and pay a higher portion of the drug cost until you reach Stage 4.

Some drug plans provide additional coverage to help lower your share of the cost of prescription drugs if you have a gap in coverage.

NOTE: If you receive Medicare Extra Help you will NOT go into the donut hole; you will stay in Stage 2, regardless of the amount of your total drug cost.

PART D COVERS
STAGE 4:
CATASTROPHIC COVERAGE

When your true out-of-pocket (TrOOP) cost reaches **$6,350** you will enter Stage 4 and receive catastrophic coverage. In this stage, you only pay a small copayment or insurance amount for the remainder of the calendar year.

Your true out-of-pocket cost includes:
- Annual deductible
- Copayments
- Coinsurance
- Discount on brand-name drugs

It does NOT include:
- Monthly premium
- Pharmacy dispensing fee
- Non-covered drugs

Annual Notice of Changes | Evidence of Coverage

In the fall, your plan will send you a printed **Annual Notice of Changes (ANOC)** about changes to your Medicare Prescription Drug plan's coverage, costs, service area, and more that will go into effect on JAN 1. Your plan will also send you an **Evidence of Coverage (EOC) notice or printed copy** with details about what your plan covers, how much you pay, and more. Review these two notices carefully to make sure your plan will still meet your needs in the coming year. If not, you may switch plans during the Annual Enrollment Period (OCT 15 - DEC 7).

Star ratings

Medicare uses a star rating to measure the quality and performance of Medicare Prescription Drug plans. The overall rating tells you about the drug plan's quality and performance in these four areas:

1. Drug plan customer service
2. Member complaints and changes in the drug plan's performance
3. Member experience with the drug plan
4. Drug safety and accuracy of drug pricing

This information is collected from:
- Member surveys
- Billing and other information that plans submit to Medicare
- Medicare's regular monitoring activities

YOUR COST

MEDICARE PART

D

MEDICARE PRESCRIPTION DRUG PLAN

YOUR COST FOR PART D (2020)

MONTHLY PREMIUM

Varies by company & plan.
Higher-income consumers may pay more.

Part D late-enrollment penalty

If you go 63 or more continuous days without having Medicare Part D or other "creditable" coverage after the last day of your Initial Enrollment Period, you may pay a penalty of 1% of the National Base Beneficiary Premium [$32.74 in 2020] times the number of full uncovered months rounded to the nearest $.10, for as long as you have Part D.

"Creditable" coverage means that the coverage is expected to pay on average as much as the standard Medicare prescription drug coverage.

Group health insurance plans from employers with 20 or more employees and unions are generally creditable.

YOUR COST FOR PART D (2020)

ANNUAL DEDUCTIBLE

Varies by company & plan.
($0 - $435/year)

If your Medicare Prescription Drug plan has an annual deductible you must pay this amount before the plan will pay its share for covered prescription drugs.

YOUR COST FOR PART D (2020)

COPAYMENT & COINSURANCE

Varies by company & plan.
Most plans group drugs into cost-sharing tiers.

Each plan decides which drugs they will cover and how much they will charge. Some drugs have a copayment (dollar amount), others have a coinsurance (percentage of the negotiated cost for that drug).

If the amount of your year-to-date total drug cost reaches **$4,020**, your plan may have a **COVERAGE GAP**. In this donut hole, you pay no more than 25% of the plan's cost for covered drugs. When your true out-of-pocket (TrOOP) cost reaches a total of **$6,350**, you automatically receive **CATASTROPHIC COVERAGE** and only pay a small copay for the remainder of the year.

On some plans, all of your drugs may be in Tier 1 and Tier 2.

On other plans, they may be in Tier 1 and Tier 3, which costs a LOT more money.

Some plans may not cover some of your drugs at all. ($$$$)

YOUR COST FOR PART D (2020)

EXTRA HELP & SPAP

A financial assistance program called **Medicare Extra Help** is available for Medicare beneficiaries who need help paying for their prescription drugs.

You *may* qualify for Extra Help if:
- You have Medicare Part A and/or Part B
- You have limited resources
- You live in one of the 50 states or the District of Columbia

You *automatically* qualify for Extra Help if:
- You have full Medicaid, or...
- Get SSI (Supplemental Security Income) benefits, or...
- Medicaid helps pay for your Part B premiums (through a Medicare Savings Program)

If you don't qualify for Extra Help:
Many states and the U.S. Virgin Islands offer help paying for Medicare Prescription Drug plan premiums and/or other drug costs. You may qualify for a **State Pharmaceutical Assistance Program (SPAP),** such as **Senior Rx/Disability Rx.**

PART D
ENROLLMENT PERIODS

You can only enroll in or make a change to a Medicare Prescription Drug plan during specific enrollment periods.

Part D Initial Enrollment Period (IEP)

If you have Medicare Part A *or* Part B, you can enroll in a Medicare Prescription Drug plan during your 7-month Initial Enrollment Period (IEP).

IF YOU DON'T HAVE PART A, AND YOU ENROLL IN PART B FOR THE FIRST TIME DURING THE GENERAL ENROLLMENT PERIOD (GEP) between JAN 1 - MAR 31, you can enroll in a drug plan between APR 1 - JUN 30. Coverage starts JULY 1.

IF YOU ARE NEWLY ELIGIBLE FOR MEDICARE BECAUSE YOU HAVE A DISABILITY AND YOU ARE UNDER 65 you may enroll in a Medicare Prescription Drug plan after you've received Social Security or Railroad Retirement Board (RRB) disability benefits for a full 24 months. You have 7 months to enroll in a plan. (Starts 3 months before your 25th month, includes the 25th month, and ends 3 months after your 25th month.) If you enroll during the 3 months before your 25th month, your coverage starts on the first day of the 25th month. If you enroll in the 25th - 28th month, your coverage begins on the first day of the month after you enroll.

IF YOU ARE ALREADY ELIGIBLE FOR MEDICARE BECAUSE YOU HAVE A DISABILITY AND YOU TURN 65, you

may use your 7-month Initial Enrollment Period (IEP) to:
- Enroll in a Medicare Prescription Drug plan
- Switch from your current Medicare Prescription Drug plan to another Medicare Prescription Drug
- Drop your Medicare Prescription Drug plan

Annual Enrollment Period (AEP) OCT 15 - DEC 7

During this enrollment period, you may:
- Enroll in a Medicare Prescription Drug plan
- Switch from one Medicare Prescription Drug plan to another Medicare Prescription Drug plan
- Drop your Medicare Prescription Drug plan

Changes go into effect on JAN 1.

Medicare Advantage Open Enrollment Period (MA-OEP) JAN 1 - MAR 31

If you are using this enrollment period to drop your Medicare Advantage plan and return to Original Medicare, you may add a Medicare Prescription Drug plan to your coverage at this time. Changes start on the first day of the month after the plan gets your request.

Medicare Advantage Open Enrollment Period: New (MA-OEP New)

You may (only) use this enrollment period to enroll in a Medicare Prescription Drug plan *if*:
- You joined a Medicare Advantage plan during your Initial Enrollment Period, *and*
- You qualified for a "3-Month Medicare Advantage Trial Period," *and*
- You are within the 3-month trial period, *and*
- You are using this enrollment period to drop your

Medicare Advantage plan and return to Original Medicare

Special Circumstances | Special Enrollment Periods (SEP)

When certain life events happen after your Initial Enrollment Period (IEP) has passed, you may be able to use a Special Enrollment Period to enroll in, switch, or drop your Medicare Prescription Drug plan. For example, you qualify for a Special Enrollment Period to enroll in a Medicare Prescription Drug plan at any time if you are eligible (or lose your eligibility) for Extra Help.

5-Star Special Enrollment Period (5-Star SEP) DEC 8 - NOV 30

If a 5-Star Medicare Advantage plan, 5-Star Cost plan, or a 5-Star Medicare Prescription Drug plan is available in your service area, you can use this Special Enrollment Period to make a one-time switch to that plan. (A 5-star rating is considered excellent. These ratings can change every year.)

MEDIGAP PLAN

a~n

AVAILABLE THROUGH PRIVATE COMPANIES

MEDICARE SUPPLEMENT INSURANCE

MEDIGAP: MEDICARE SUPPLEMENT INSURANCE

Medicare Supplement Insurance, called Medigap, is available from private companies to *supplement* Original Medicare. These plans help you pay for some of the costs that Original Medicare does not pay for, such as your copays, coinsurance, etc. Some plans also cover additional services that are not covered by Original Medicare, such as foreign travel emergency care.

All Medigap plans must be clearly identified as "Medicare Supplement Insurance" and must follow federal and state laws that are in place to protect you. These plans are available in all states and Washington D.C. (Massachusetts, Minnesota, and Wisconsin have their own standardized Medigap plans.)

To be eligible for Medigap you must be enrolled in Medicare Part A *and* Part B. If you do not enroll during your Medigap Open Enrollment Period you may be required to go through medical underwriting, which means that the insurer may take a close look at your medical history, pre-existing conditions, and other risk factors when reviewing your application. As a result of this you could be denied coverage or have a waiting period. Some states allow special exceptions and/or have additional rules. See "Medigap Enrollment Periods."

Each company decides which Medigap plans it wants to sell. They are generally distinguished by their plan letter: **a, b, c, d, f, g, k, l, m**, and **n**. (Companies are not required to offer every plan in every state, however, all Medigap plans are required to offer the same basic benefits.)

Medigap plans that cover the Part B deductible can no longer be sold to people who are newly eligible for Medicare on or after 01/01/2020. Those who already have **Plan c** and **Plan f** are grandfathered in.

In some states, some insurers offer a Medigap plan called Medicare SELECT. These plans generally have lower monthly premiums. Much like an HMO, members must use in-network doctors and facilities, except in emergencies. Other than that, they function like a standard Medigap plan. (If you buy a Medicare SELECT plan, you have the right to change your mind within 12 months and switch to a standard Medigap plan.)

While federal law does not require insurance companies to sell Medigap plans to people under 65, in some states there are state laws that require insurance companies to offer at least one kind of Medigap plan to people with Medicare under the age of 65. Some provide the right to buy a Medigap plan to ALL people under 65 who are eligible for Medicare; others only provide it for those under 65 who are eligible for Medicare because of a disability or ESRD. (Not all states offer a Medigap plan to those with ESRD.)

NOTE: Medicare Supplement Insurance cannot be used to help you pay for a Medicare Advantage Plan's out-of-pocket costs. In fact, it is illegal for anyone to sell you a Medigap plan If you're enrolled in a Medicare Advantage plan unless you are switching back to Original Medicare prior to your policy's effective date.

There are (10) standard Medigap plans.

Let's take a look at each of these plans to see what they cover.

MEDIGAP (2020)

Plan a

Your cost varies by company.

100% COVERAGE
- Part A coinsurance and hospital costs up to an additional 365 days after Medicare benefits are used up
- Part A hospice care coinsurance/copay
- Part B coinsurance/copay
- Blood (first 3 pints)

NO COVERAGE
- Part A deductible
- Part A skilled nursing (SNF) coinsurance
- Part B deductible
- Part B excess charge
- Foreign travel exchange

ANNUAL OUT-OF-POCKET LIMIT (n/a)

MEDIGAP (2020)

Plan b

Your cost varies by company.

100% COVERAGE
- Part A coinsurance and hospital costs up to an additional 365 days after Medicare benefits are used up
- Part A deductible
- Part A hospice care coinsurance/copay
- Part B coinsurance/copay
- Blood (first 3 pints)

NO COVERAGE
- Part A skilled nursing (SNF) coinsurance
- Part B deductible
- Part B excess charge
- Foreign travel exchange

ANNUAL OUT-OF-POCKET LIMIT (n/a)

MEDIGAP (2020)

Plan c

Your cost varies by company.

100% COVERAGE
- Part A coinsurance and hospital costs up to an additional 365 days after Medicare benefits are used up
- Part A deductible
- Part A hospice care coinsurance/copay
- Part A skilled nursing (SNF) coinsurance
- Part B coinsurance/copay
- Part B deductible
- Blood (first 3 pints)

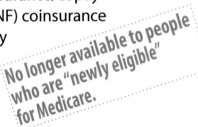
No longer available to people who are "newly eligible" for Medicare.

80% COVERAGE
- Foreign travel exchange (up to plan limits). This covers medical expenses after you meet the $250 annual deductible, and foreign travel emergency care (if required during the first 60 days of your trip) and Medicare does not pay the cost. Lifetime benefit maximum: $50,000.

NO COVERAGE
- Part B excess charge

ANNUAL OUT-OF-POCKET LIMIT (n/a)

MEDIGAP (2020)

Plan d

Your cost varies by company.

100% COVERAGE

- Part A coinsurance and hospital costs up to an additional 365 days after Medicare benefits are used up
- Part A deductible
- Part A hospice care coinsurance/copay
- Part A skilled nursing (SNF) coinsurance
- Part B coinsurance/copay
- Blood (first 3 pints)

80% COVERAGE

- Foreign travel exchange (up to plan limits). This covers medical expenses after you meet the $250 annual deductible, and foreign travel emergency care (if required during the first 60 days of your trip) and Medicare does not pay the cost. Lifetime benefit maximum: $50,000.

NO COVERAGE

- Part B deductible
- Part B excess charge

ANNUAL OUT-OF-POCKET LIMIT (n/a)

MEDIGAP (2020)

Plan f*

Your cost varies by company.

100% COVERAGE

- Part A coinsurance and hospital costs up to an additional 365 days after Medicare benefits are used up
- Part A deductible
- Part A hospice care coinsurance/copay
- Part A skilled nursing (SNF) coinsurance
- Part B coinsurance/copay
- Part B deductible
- Part B excess charge
- Blood (first 3 pints)

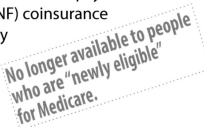

No longer available to people who are "newly eligible" for Medicare.

80% COVERAGE

- Foreign travel exchange (up to plan limits). This covers medical expenses after you meet the $250 annual deductible, and foreign travel emergency care (if required during the first 60 days of your trip) and Medicare does not pay the cost. Lifetime benefit maximum: $50,000.

ANNUAL OUT-OF-POCKET LIMIT (n/a)

*There is also a High-Deductible Plan f

(Only available to those who were eligible for Medicare BEFORE 1/1/2020. You pay for Medicare-covered costs up to **$2,340** before your plan pays anything.)

MEDIGAP (2020)

Plan g*

Your cost varies by company.

100% COVERAGE
- Part A coinsurance and hospital costs up to an additional 365 days after Medicare benefits are used up
- Part A deductible
- Part A hospice care coinsurance/copay
- Part A skilled nursing (SNF) coinsurance
- Part B coinsurance/copay
- Part B excess charge
- Blood (first 3 pints)

80% COVERAGE
- Foreign travel exchange (up to plan limits). This covers medical expenses after you meet the $250 annual deductible, and foreign travel emergency care (if required during the first 60 days of your trip) and Medicare does not pay the cost. Lifetime benefit maximum: $50,000.

NO COVERAGE
- Part B deductible

ANNUAL OUT-OF-POCKET LIMIT (n/a)

*There is also a High-Deductible Plan g
(Only available to those who are newly eligible for Medicare ON or AFTER 1/1/2020. You pay for Medicare-covered costs up to **$2,340** before your plan pays anything.)

MEDIGAP (2020)

Plan k

Your cost varies by company.

100% COVERAGE
· Part A coinsurance and hospital costs up to an additional 365 days after Medicare benefits are used up

50% COVERAGE
· Part A deductible
· Part A hospice care coinsurance/copay
· Part A skilled nursing (SNF) coinsurance
· Part B coinsurance/copay
· Blood (first 3 pints)

NO COVERAGE
· Part B deductible
· Part B excess charge
· Foreign travel exchange

ANNUAL OUT-OF-POCKET LIMIT: $5,880
After you meet this limit and your annual Part B deductible, your Medigap plan pays 100%.

MEDIGAP (2020)

Plan I

Your cost varies by company.

100% COVERAGE
- Part A coinsurance and hospital costs up to an additional 365 days after Medicare benefits are used up

75% COVERAGE
- Part A deductible
- Part A hospice care coinsurance/copay
- Part A skilled nursing (SNF) coinsurance
- Part B coinsurance/copay
- Blood (first 3 pints)

NO COVERAGE
- Part B deductible
- Part B excess charge
- Foreign travel exchange

ANNUAL OUT-OF-POCKET LIMIT: $2,940
After you meet this limit and your annual Part B deductible, your Medigap plan pays 100%.

MEDIGAP (2020)

Plan m

Your cost varies by company.

100% COVERAGE
- Part A coinsurance and hospital costs up to an additional 365 days after Medicare benefits are used up
- Part A hospice care coinsurance/copay
- Part A skilled nursing (SNF) coinsurance
- Part B coinsurance/copay
- Blood (first 3 pints)

80% COVERAGE
- Foreign travel exchange (up to plan limits). This covers medical expenses after you meet the $250 annual deductible, and foreign travel emergency care (if required during the first 60 days of your trip) and Medicare does not pay the cost. Lifetime benefit maximum: $50,000.

50% COVERAGE
- Part A deductible

NO COVERAGE
- Part B deductible
- Part B excess charge

ANNUAL OUT-OF-POCKET LIMIT (n/a)

MEDIGAP (2020)

Plan n

Your cost varies by company.

100% COVERAGE
· Part A coinsurance and hospital costs up to an additional 365 days after Medicare benefits are used up
· Part A deductible
· Part A hospice care coinsurance/copay
· Part A skilled nursing (SNF) coinsurance
· Part B coinsurance/copay, except for a copay of up to $20 for some office visits and up to $50 for E.R. visits that don't result in inpatient admission
· Blood (first 3 pints)

80% COVERAGE
· Foreign travel exchange (up to plan limits). This covers medical expenses after you meet the $250 annual deductible, and foreign travel emergency care (if required during the first 60 days of your trip) and Medicare does not pay the cost. Lifetime benefit maximum: $50,000.

NO COVERAGE
· Part B deductible
· Part B excess charge

ANNUAL OUT-OF-POCKET LIMIT (n/a)

Can I switch to another Medigap plan?

Yes, but you will most likely be required to go through medical underwriting *unless:*
1. You are still within your 6-month Medigap Open Enrollment Period, *or*
2. You have a special circumstance that qualifies you for a Special Enrollment Period, *or*
3. You have guaranteed issue rights, *or*
4. You live in a state that does not allow companies to use medical underwriting for Medigap.

If you would like to change insurance companies:
1. Call the new insurance company and arrange to submit an application. They will ask you to promise to cancel your current policy. But don't cancel it yet!
2. If your application is accepted, call your current insurance company and ask them how to submit a request to stop your coverage. But don't cancel it yet! If your application is declined, you can simply keep the policy you have, submit an application to another insurance company, or ask your current insurer if you can switch to another policy that they offer.
3. When your new policy arrives you will get a "30-Day Free Look Period." During this one month, you must pay for BOTH policies. Don't cancel your first policy until you know with absolute certainty that you want to keep the second policy, because once you've canceled a policy you cannot get it back!
4. Decide which policy you want to keep and cancel the other one.

YOUR COST

MEDIGAP PLAN

a~n

MEDICARE SUPPLEMENT INSURANCE

YOUR COST FOR A MEDIGAP PLAN

Although all Medigap plans are standardized, **your cost for identical plans can vary widely by company.**

Are you comparing (red) apples to (red) apples?

While it may be tempting to buy whichever Medigap plan has the lowest premium, there are several other factors that you should take into consideration when comparing plans, such as:

Do they offer a discount?

Some companies offer discounts to non-smokers, married people, households with a specified number of residents, and other criteria. Be sure to read the fine print carefully to see if the discount decreases over time. If so, even though the plan is not technically increasing as you get older, you still may be paying more out-of-pocket as you age. And sometimes it's cheaper, in the long run, to buy a fitness club membership yourself than to choose a Medigap plan that includes a "free" fitness club membership.

Do they have similar histories of rate increases?

While this has no real bearing on what the insurance company will do with their premiums in the future, it's good to know what your experience would have been like if you had purchased this plan a few years ago.

Do they have the same plan letter?

Make sure you are comparing plans with the same plan letter, such as a **Medigap Plan g** to a **Medigap Plan g**.

Do they use the same rating (pricing) method?

There are three different rating methods that an insurance company can use to set the price for a Medigap policy.

COMMUNITY-RATED POLICY

Everyone who purchases a community-rated policy pays the same premium, regardless of their age. Your premium will not increase due to getting older, but will likely increase due to inflation and other factors.

ISSUE-AGE-RATED POLICY

Your premium is based on your age at the time of purchase. (When the policy is "issued" to you.) Your premium will not increase due to getting older, but will likely increase due to inflation and other factors.

ATTAINED-AGE-RATED POLICY

Your premium is based on your current age. (The age you have "attained.") Therefore, it will increase as you get older, and will likely increase due to inflation and other factors, as well.

Make sure you are comparing plans with the same rating method, such as an issue-rated policy to an issue-rated policy.

Do they have the same financial rating?

A carrier with a B+ or higher rating will typically be more established and have more financial stability.

MEDIGAP ENROLLMENT PERIODS

Those who are 65 years of age or older and enrolled in Medicare Part B may apply for a Medigap plan at any time of the year. The best time to enroll is during the Medigap Open Enrollment Period.

Medigap Open Enrollment Period (OEP)

This 6-month period begins the first day of the month in which you are 65 years of age or older and you have Part B. During this time you have **"guaranteed issue rights."** You can buy any Medigap plan the company sells in your market for the same price as someone of the same age who has no pre-existing health conditions. Your application cannot be declined.

If you miss the Medigap Open Enrollment Period and do not qualify for a Special Enrollment Period, most insurers will require you to go through medical underwriting to determine your insurability (unless your state allows special exceptions). If you have a pre-existing condition, the insurance company can:

- Decline your application.
- Accept your application but restrict your coverage with a 6-month "pre-existing condition waiting period." During this time, your pre-existing condition will only be covered by Medicare; you will have to pay the full coinsurance-copayment amount.
- Charge you a higher premium.

So, if you have a chronic or critical illness and want to

purchase a Medigap plan, make sure to use this enrollment period (or a Special Enrollment Period, if you qualify) to ensure that you are guaranteed coverage at no additional cost and with no waiting period.

Special Circumstances | Special Enrollment Periods (SEP)

If you are 65 years of age or older, and certain life events happen after your 6-month Medigap Open Enrollment Period has passed, you may be able to qualify for a guaranteed-issue Medigap plan if you apply within 63 days of (when):

- Through no fault of your own, you lose an employer-sponsored insurance plan that supplemented your Medicare. This Special Enrollment Period begins 60 days before your current plan expires.
- You move out of the area that's covered by a Medigap plan.
- Your insurer goes bankrupt or misrepresents a provision in your plan.
- You disenroll from a Medicare Advantage plan (that you had enrolled in when you first became eligible for Medicare) within 12 months of enrolling in it.

NOTE: Some states have additional Medigap rules.

For example:

- **CALIFORNIA:** Anyone who is enrolled in a Medigap plan can use the "Birthday Rule" to switch to any other Medigap plan with equal or lesser benefits offered by any company during their birth month with a guaranteed issue. You can apply up to 30 days before and after your birthday, which gives you a total of 61 days to make a change to your plan.

- **CONNECTICUT:** All Medigap plans are available on a guaranteed issue basis with no medical underwriting. However, if an applicant has no prior creditable coverage or has experienced a gap in coverage, a pre-existing condition limitation may apply. Premium rates may not be based on your age, gender, or health status.
- **MAINE:** Each insurer must designate a one-month guaranteed issue period each year when any applicant will be accepted in **Medigap Plan a.** Insurers must also offer you a guaranteed issue plan if you apply for a Medigap plan within 90 days of losing coverage from an individual health insurance plan, a group health plan through your employer, or MaineCares. (Some restrictions apply.) And anyone with a Medigap plan who has never had a gap in coverage of 90 or more days since Open Enrollment can switch to a plan with equal or lesser benefits from any insurer at any time of the year with guaranteed issue.
- **MISSOURI:** Anyone with a Medigap plan can use the "Anniversary Guaranteed Issue Period" to switch to another Medigap plan with guaranteed issue. You have from 30 days before your enrollment anniversary until 30 days after it to make a change.
- **NEW YORK:** All Medigap plans are guaranteed issue. If you have a pre-existing condition, insurers are required to reduce the waiting period by the number of days that you were covered under some form of "creditable" coverage, so long as there were no breaks in coverage of more than 63 calendar days.
- **OREGON:** Anyone who is enrolled in a Medigap plan can use the "Birthday Rule" to switch to any other Medigap plan with equal or lesser benefits that are offered by any company during their birth month with a guaranteed issue. It starts on your birthday and ends 30 days later.

OTHER MEDICARE HEALTH PLANS

Medicare Cost plan

Medicare Cost plans are only available in certain areas of the country. In some ways, they are similar to a Medicare Advantage plan; in other ways they are very different.

- You can enroll in a Medicare Cost plan even if you only have Part B.
- You can join any time the plan is accepting new members.
- You can leave the plan at any time and return to Original Medicare.
- You have the option of going to in-network or out-of-network providers. When you go out-of-network your services are covered by Original Medicare and you pay the Part A and Part B deductibles and coinsurance.
- If the plan includes prescription drug coverage you can choose to get your prescriptions from the plan *or* enroll in a Medicare Prescription Drug plan.

Another type of Medicare Cost plan only provides coverage for Part B services; it never includes Part D. (Part A services are covered through Original Medicare.) These plans are either sponsored by employer or union group health plans or offered by companies that don't provide Part A services.

PACE (Programs of All-Inclusive Care for the Elderly)

PACE is a Medicare/Medicaid program that helps people "who need a nursing home level of care" to get the health care services they need in their community, such as in their own home or at a PACE center, so they don't have to be confined to a nursing home or other care facility.

Those who are enrolled in PACE have a team of health care professionals who take the time to get to know you, and work closely with you and your family to make sure you are getting the level of coordinated care and services you need.

To be eligible for coverage, you must be:
- 55 years of age, or older
- Certified by your state as needing a nursing home level of care
- Able to live safely in the community with the help of PACE services (at the time of enrollment)
- Living in the service area of a PACE organization

If you have MEDICARE AND MEDICAID there is no monthly premium for the long-term care portion of your PACE benefit.

If you have MEDICARE ONLY you will be charged a monthly premium to cover the long-term care portion of your PACE benefits plus a premium for Medicare Part D prescription drugs. There is no deductible or copayment for any service, care, or drug approved by your health care team.

Medicare Demonstrations and Pilot Programs

Medicare periodically conducts research studies to test improvements in their coverage, payment, and quality of care. These special projects usually run for a limited time, in specific areas, for a specific group of people. Call 1-800-MEDICARE to get more information on these programs.

WHICH MEDICARE PLAN IS BEST FOR ME?

Let's review your options.

If you have Original Medicare Part A and Part B (only):

- You can go to any hospital, doctor, or provider in the U.S. that accepts Medicare.
- Part A covers your inpatient hospital stay, skilled nursing care in a skilled nursing facility, home health care, and hospice care services. Your out-of-pocket costs include a monthly premium ($0 for most people), hospital deductible, hospital coinsurance, and skilled nursing facility coinsurance.
- Part B covers medically necessary services, mental health care, preventative and screening services, and durable medical equipment. Your Part B out-of-pocket cost includes a monthly premium, annual deductible, medical copayment, and medical coinsurance.
- Medicare will NOT cover outpatient prescription drugs, acupuncture, routine dental care (cleanings, exams, X-rays, or dentures), routine vision care (exams for glasses/contact lenses), routine hearing care (exams for hearing aids), routine foot care, or routine preventative physical exams.
- There is NO ANNUAL LIMIT on your Part A and Part B out-of-pocket costs which can potentially add up to a financially catastrophic amount of money.

Fortunately, you have other options. Medicare plans are also available through private companies to help you fill some of the gaps in coverage and provide financial protection.

3 Ways to Fill the Gaps and Minimize Your Financial Risk:

OPTION 1

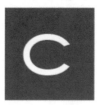

Enroll in a Medicare Advantage Plan
that includes a Medicare Prescription Drug Plan.

OPTION 2

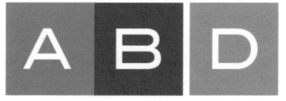

Stay in Original Medicare.
Add a Prescription Drug Plan.

OPTION 3

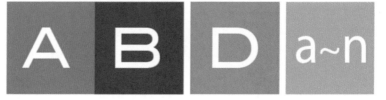

Stay in Original Medicare.
Add a Prescription Drug Plan
and a Medigap Plan.

The option that's best for you may be very different from the option that's best for your spouse or friend because we all have different needs, preferences, and priorities.

OPTION 1:

Enroll in a Medicare Advantage plan (Part C) that includes a Medicare Prescription Drug plan (Part D). These plans provide all your Medicare Part A and Part B benefits, plus (usually) some extra coverage, such as routine dental, vision, and hearing care, and more. All plans have a maximum out-of-pocket limit (MOOP) to provide you with a financial safety net. Most plans have a network of providers. PPO plans will generally allow you to go out-of-network to any doctor or facility that accepts Medicare, for a higher cost.

OPTION 2:

Stay in Original Medicare (Part A and Part B) and add a Medicare Prescription Drug plan (Part D) to your coverage. With this option there's NO LIMIT on how much your Part A and Part B out-of-pocket costs can add up; you have no financial safety net (unless you receive financial assistance from the government, such as Medicaid). You can go to any doctor or facility in the U.S. that accepts Medicare.

OPTION 3:

Stay in Original Medicare (Part A and Part B) and add a Medicare Prescription Drug plan (Part D) *plus* Medigap (Plan a~n). Part D helps you fill the drug coverage gap; Medigap provides you with a financial safety net by helping you cover some of your Part A and Part B out-of-pocket costs. You can go to any doctor or facility that accepts Medicare.

Now it's time to meet with an agent.

Working with an agent who is familiar with Medicare plans that are available in your market will save you an enormous amount of time and frustration! Best of all, licensed agents generally do NOT charge a fee for this service! Agents earn a commission from insurance companies for explaining a plan's benefits and costs to you, answering your questions, confirming your eligibility, and submitting your application.

The best way to find a good agent is through referrals from friends, family, coworkers, neighbors, or people in your church, club, or organization.

An agent who genuinely cares about their clients:
- Asks if you *understand* what Medicare covers and doesn't cover before launching into a sales presentation.
- Does a quick needs analysis (ask questions) to evaluate your individual needs, preferences, and priorities.
- Educates you about the difference between a Medicare Advantage plan and a Medicare Supplement Insurance plan, and then has YOU choose which one you'd like to enroll in.
- Gives you options, and doesn't just sell you a plan.
- Reaches out to you during the Annual Enrollment Period to review upcoming changes to your plan's copays, prescription drug costs, etc., and make sure your plan still fits your needs well for the coming year. If not, they will help you find a plan that fits your needs better.
- Answers your phone calls in a timely manner
- Is always happy to help you resolve issues if/when they arise.

FINANCIAL ASSISTANCE PROGRAMS

The following financial assistance programs are available for those who meet certain income and resource limits.

Medicaid

This joint federal and state program helps some people with limited income and resources with medical costs. Medicaid offers benefits not normally covered by Medicare, like nursing home care and personal care services. Each state has different rules about eligibility and applying for Medicaid.

Medicare Extra Help

If you have limited resources and income, this Medicare program may help you pay for your Medicare Prescription Drug plan costs. (You must reside in one of the 50 states or the District of Columbia.)

Medicare Savings Programs (MSP)

This state program may help you pay for Medicare premiums, deductibles, coinsurance, copayments, and the cost of prescription drugs.

- **Qualified Medicare Beneficiary (QMB)**
  Helps pay for your Part A premiums, Part B premiums, deductibles, copayments, and coinsurance.
- **Specified Low-Income Medicare Beneficiary (SLMB)**
  Helps pay for Part B premiums only.
- **Qualifying Individual (QI or QI-1)**
  Helps pay for Part B premiums only. Funding is limited; applications are granted on a first-come, first-served basis.

- **Qualified Disabled & Working Individual (QDWI)**
Helps pay for Part A premiums only.

NOTE: Those who qualify for a QMB, SLMB, or QI Medicare Savings Program automatically qualify for Extra Help.

PACE (Programs of All-inclusive Care for the Elderly)

This Medicare/Medicaid program provides comprehensive medical and social services to certain frail, community-dwelling elderly individuals.

Programs for people in U.S. territories

Financial assistance is available in Puerto Rico, U.S. Virgin Islands, Guam, Northern Mariana Islands, and American Samoa for those who need help paying for Medicare costs. These programs vary by territory.

State Pharmaceutical Assistance Program (SPAP)

Many states offer help paying for prescription drugs.

Supplemental Social Security Income (SSI)

This program pays benefits to disabled adults (and children) who have little or no income and provides cash to meet basic needs for food, clothing, and shelter. It also pays benefits to people 65 and older without disabilities who meet the financial limits.

TRAVELING WITH MEDICARE INSURANCE

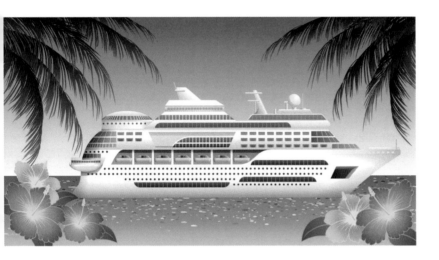

"Am I covered by Medicare when I travel?"

That depends. Where are you going? And which Medicare insurance plan do you have?

If you are planning to take a cruise, it's important to know that you are only covered by Original Medicare if the ship is in U.S. waters, and if the physician treating you is legally allowed to provide medical care on a cruise ship. Once your ship is six hours away from the nearest U.S. port, you are in the country of whatever flag is flying on the mainmast of your ship, and most cruise ships are registered in a foreign country. So, unless you are enrolled in a Medicare plan that covers foreign travel, it may offer little or no protection or reimbursement for the costs of any medical treatments received on board a cruise ship.

If you have Original Medicare (Part A and Part B) only:

If you get hurt or sick while traveling *within* the 50 states, the District of Columbia, Puerto Rico, U.S. Virgin Islands, Guam, Northern Mariana Islands, or American Samoa, you can go to ANY doctor, hospital, or other facility that accepts Medicare.

Medicare generally does NOT cover health care if you travel *outside* the United States and its territories, except in rare circumstances, such as:

- If you're in the U.S. when a medical emergency happens and a hospital in a foreign country is closer than the hospital that can treat your injuries.
- If you have a medical emergency while traveling by the most direct route from Alaska to another state, you can be treated in a Canadian hospital if it's closer than the nearest U.S. hospital.
- If you live in the U.S. and a foreign hospital is closer to your home than the nearest U.S. hospital that can treat you, you can go to the foreign hospital, whether you have an emergency or not.

If you have a Medigap plan:

Since Medigap plans supplement Original Medicare, you can go to ANY doctor, hospital, or other facility that accepts Medicare while traveling *within* the U.S. and its territories, and outside the U.S. in rare circumstances.

Medigap plans **c, d, f, g, m,** and **n** cover foreign travel emergency care *if it begins during the first 60 days of your trip and if Medicare doesn't otherwise cover the care.* These plans pay 80% of the billed charges for certain medically necessary emergency care outside the U.S. after you meet a $250 deductible for the year ($50,000 lifetime limit).

If you have a Medicare Advantage plan:

All Medicare Advantage plans cover emergency and urgently needed medical care in the United States and its territories. When you are outside of your plan's service area you should go to the nearest hospital emergency room for treatment.

Some Medicare Advantage plans provide global coverage, as well. If yours does and you receive medical care abroad, be sure to get an itemized copy of the bill *written in English* to submit to your plan for reimbursement when you get home.

NOTE: If you plan to do a lot of traveling, and there's a chance that you'll be away from home for an extended period of time, here's something important to know: MOST Medicare Advantage plans will automatically disenroll you from your plan and place you back in Original Medicare if you travel outside of your service area continuously for more than 6 months! If you are disenrolled from a plan that includes prescription drug coverage you may incur a Part D late enrollment penalty if you go 63 or more continuous days without having Medicare Part D or other "creditable" drug coverage.

Ask your agent to help you review your Medicare Advantage plan's rules and restrictions regarding being out of your service area continuously for six months or more. If another plan fits your needs better, you can switch plans during the upcoming Annual Enrollment Period, from OCT 15 to DEC 7.

Some Medicare Advantage plans have a travel benefit that allows you to travel continuously outside of your service area for up to 12 months. Only certain areas may be covered unless you need emergency or urgent medical care, and/or you may pay more to see providers outside of your plan's network.

"Should I buy travel insurance?"

Travel insurance policies offered by cruise lines and tour groups generally have *significant restrictions and limitations.* To get the best rates and coverage, it's best to buy a policy from a reputable insurance company that works with all of the major carriers.

There are many different types of Travel Insurance plans to choose from.

Trip Protection

Trip protection is a combination of benefits which may include coverage for trip cancellation, trip interruption, travel delays, emergency medical, emergency medical evacuation, baggage protection, baggage delay, and 24-hour emergency assistance services.

Travel Medical/International Medical

Travel Medical Insurance reimburses you for emergency medical expenses incurred when you are traveling or living in a foreign country. Maximum coverage levels can be substantial enough to cover major medical expenses such as emergency surgery and extended hospital stays. Plans usually include coverage for emergency medical evacuation, reunion, repatriation of remains, accidental death and dismemberment (AD&D), and other 24/7 travel assistance services.

Emergency Medical Evacuation

Depending on the plan, emergency medical evacuation covers the cost of transporting a seriously injured or ill person to the nearest adequate medical facility, a hospital near home, or the hospital of his/her choice.

Accidental Death & Dismemberment

Flight accident insurance, common carrier accident insurance, and/or 24-hour accidental death insurance pays you or your beneficiary a lump sum benefit when an accident results in your death, loss of a limb, or loss of your eyesight.

Global Risk

These plans specifically cover high-risk situations such as business travel to high-risk or war-risk countries. Coverages available include travel medical insurance, emergency medical evacuation, and accidental death and dismemberment insurance with no exclusions for incidents involving acts of war or terrorism. This category is also where you'll find kidnap and ransom insurance, Defense Base Act insurance, and high-limit accidental death and dismemberment.

Annual Multi-Trip

Designed for year-round peace of mind for people who love to travel, annual multi-trip travel insurance plans provide coverage for all of your trips throughout the year. (Maximum trip length of 30 to 180 days per trip depending on the plan.)

Group Travel

If your group consists of 10 or more traveling on the same trip itinerary, a group travel insurance plan may be your most economical choice! Many group plans are not age-banded; premiums vary according to the trip cost per person. Comprehensive group protection plans include trip cancellation, travel interruption and delay, emergency medical, emergency medical evacuation, lost or delayed baggage and more. You can also purchase coverage for just medical and/or medical evacuation.

A NOTE
FROM THE AUTHOR

I welcome your questions, comments, suggestions, and of course, testimonials! I'd love to know if this book helped you to understand Medicare insurance better.
Email: Linda@HeartToHeartInsurance.com
Website: HeartToHeartInsurance.com

Would you kindly take a few minutes to write a short review of this book for me on Amazon? This will help others find it when they are searching online for information about Medicare. Go to: https://amzn.to/32vbz8k

Thank you so much!
From the heart - Linda

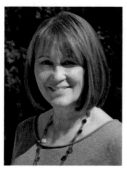

Linda A. Bell is an Independent Life & Health Insurance Broker and Field Underwriter in Las Vegas, Nevada. She is also an Artist, Photographer, and Creative Consultant.

To learn more about Linda, please visit:
HeartToHeartStudio.com

Made in the USA
Columbia, SC
17 January 2021